ENDOMETRIOSIS COOKBOOK

MAIN COURSE - 60+ Breakfast, Lunch, Dinner and Dessert Recipes to treat Endometriosis

TABLE OF CONTENTS

purposes solely, and is universal as so. The presentation of the information is without contract or any type of guarantee assurance.

The trademarks that are used are without any consent, and the publication of the trademark is without permission or backing by the trademark owner. All trademarks and brands within this book are for clarifying purposes only and are the owned by the owners themselves, not affiliated with this document.

Introduction

Endometriosis recipes for personal enjoyment but also for family enjoyment. You will love them for sure for how easy it is to prepare them.

ACAI PANCAKES

Serves: *4*

Prep Time: *10*   Minutes

Cook Time: *20*   Minutes

Total Time: *30*   Minutes

INGREDIENTS

- 1 cup whole wheat flour
- ¼ tsp baking soda
- ¼ tsp baking powder
- 1 cup acai
- 2 eggs
- 1 cup milk

DIRECTIONS

1. In a bowl combine all ingredients together and mix well
2. In a skillet heat olive oil

3. Pour ¼ of the batter and cook each pancake for 1-2 minutes per side

4. When ready remove from heat and serve

Serves: *4*

Prep Time: *10*   Minutes

Cook Time: *30*   Minutes

Total Time: *40*   Minutes

INGREDIENTS

- 1 cup whole wheat flour
- ¼ tsp baking soda
- ¼ tsp baking powder
- 1 cup akee
- 2 eggs
- 1 cup milk

DIRECTIONS

1. In a bowl combine all ingredients together and mix well
2. In a skillet heat olive oil
3. Pour ¼ of the batter and cook each pancake for 1-2 minutes per side
4. When ready remove from heat and serve

Serves: **4**
Prep Time: **10**   Minutes

Cook Time: **20**   Minutes

Total Time: **30**   Minutes

INGREDIENTS

- 1 cup whole wheat flour
- ¼ tsp baking soda
- ¼ tsp baking powder
- 1 cup mashed apple
- 2 eggs
- 1 cup milk

DIRECTIONS

1. In a bowl combine all ingredients together and mix well
2. In a skillet heat olive oil
3. Pour ¼ of the batter and cook each pancake for 1-2 minutes per side
4. When ready remove from heat and serve

Serves: *4*
Prep Time: *10* Minutes

Cook Time: *20* Minutes

Total Time: *30* Minutes

INGREDIENTS

- 1 cup whole wheat flour
- ¼ tsp baking soda
- ¼ tsp baking powder
- 1 cup avocado
- 2 eggs
- 1 cup milk

DIRECTIONS

1. In a bowl combine all ingredients together and mix well
2. In a skillet heat olive oil
3. Pour ¼ of the batter and cook each pancake for 1-2 minutes per side
4. When ready remove from heat and serve

Serves: *4*
Prep Time: *10*   Minutes

Cook Time: *30*   Minutes

Total Time: *40*   Minutes

INGREDIENTS

- 1 cup whole wheat flour
- ¼ tsp baking soda
- ¼ tsp baking powder
- 2 eggs
- 1 cup milk

DIRECTIONS

1. In a bowl combine all ingredients together and mix well
2. In a skillet heat olive oil
3. Pour ¼ of the batter and cook each pancake for 1-2 minutes per side
4. When ready remove from heat and serve

Serves:	*8-12*
Prep Time:	*10* Minutes
Cook Time:	*20* Minutes
Total Time:	*30* Minutes

INGREDIENTS

- 2 eggs
- 1 tablespoon olive oil
- 1 cup milk
- 2 cups whole wheat flour
- 1 tsp baking soda
- ¼ tsp baking soda
- 1 tsp ginger
- 1 tsp cinnamon
- ¼ cup molasses

DIRECTIONS

1. In a bowl combine all dry ingredients
2. In another bowl combine all dry ingredients

3. Combine wet and dry ingredients together

4. Pour mixture into 8-12 prepared muffin cups, fill
    2/3 of the cups

5. Bake for 18-20 minutes at 375 F

6. When ready remove from the oven and serve

Serves: *8-12*
Prep Time: *10*   Minutes

Cook Time: *20*   Minutes

Total Time: *30*   Minutes

INGREDIENTS

- **2 eggs**
- **1 tablespoon olive oil**
- **1 cup milk**
- **2 cups whole wheat flour**
- **1 tsp baking soda**
- **¼ tsp baking soda**
- **1 tsp cinnamon**
- **1 cup blackberry**

DIRECTIONS

1. **In a bowl combine all dry ingredients**
2. **In another bowl combine all dry ingredients**
3. **Combine wet and dry ingredients together**

4. Pour mixture into 8-12 prepared muffin cups, fill
    2/3 of the cups

5. Bake for 18-20 minutes at 375 F

6. When ready remove from the oven and serve

CHERRY MUFFINS

Serves: *8-12*
Prep Time: *10*   Minutes

Cook Time: *20*   Minutes

Total Time: *30*   Minutes

INGREDIENTS

- 2 eggs
- 1 tablespoon olive oil
- 1 cup milk
- 2 cups whole wheat flour
- 1 tsp baking soda
- ¼ tsp baking soda
- 1 tsp cinnamon
- 1 cup cherries

DIRECTIONS

1. In a bowl combine all dry ingredients
2. In another bowl combine all dry ingredients
3. Combine wet and dry ingredients together

4. Pour mixture into 8-12 prepared muffin cups, fill 2/3 of the cups

5. Bake for 18-20 minutes at 375 F

6. When ready remove from the oven and serve

Serves: *8-12*

Prep Time: *10*   Minutes

Cook Time: *20*   Minutes

Total Time: *30*   Minutes

INGREDIENTS

- 2 eggs
- 1 tablespoon olive oil
- 1 cup milk
- 2 cups whole wheat flour
- 1 tsp baking soda
- ¼ tsp baking soda
- 1 tsp cinnamon
- 1 cup coconut flakes

DIRECTIONS

1. In a bowl combine all dry ingredients
2. In another bowl combine all dry ingredients
3. Combine wet and dry ingredients together

4. Pour mixture into 8-12 prepared muffin cups, fill 2/3 of the cups

5. Bake for 18-20 minutes at 375 F

6. When ready remove from the oven and serve

Serves: *8-12*
Prep Time: *10*   Minutes

Cook Time: *20*   Minutes

Total Time: *30*   Minutes

INGREDIENTS

- 2 eggs
- 1 tablespoon olive oil
- 1 cup milk
- 2 cups whole wheat flour
- 1 tsp baking soda
- ¼ tsp baking soda
- 1 tsp cinnamon
- 1 cup chocolate chips

DIRECTIONS

1. In a bowl combine all dry ingredients
2. In another bowl combine all dry ingredients
3. Combine wet and dry ingredients together

4. Pour mixture into 8-12 prepared muffin cups, fill 2/3 of the cups

5. Bake for 18-20 minutes at 375 F

6. When ready remove from the oven and serve

Serves: *8-12*
Prep Time: *10*   Minutes

Cook Time: *20*   Minutes

Total Time: *30*   Minutes

INGREDIENTS

- 2 eggs
- 1 tablespoon olive oil
- 1 cup milk
- 2 cups whole wheat flour
- 1 tsp baking soda
- ¼ tsp baking soda
- 1 tsp cinnamon
- 1 cup dates

DIRECTIONS

1. In a bowl combine all dry ingredients
2. In another bowl combine all dry ingredients
3. Combine wet and dry ingredients together

4. Pour mixture into 8-12 prepared muffin cups, fill
    2/3 of the cups

5. Bake for 18-20 minutes at 375 F

6. When ready remove from the oven and serve

Serves: *1*
Prep Time: *5* Minutes

Cook Time: *10* Minutes

Total Time: *15* Minutes

INGREDIENTS

- 2 eggs
- ¼ tsp salt
- ¼ tsp black pepper
- 1 tablespoon olive oil
- ¼ cup cheese
- ¼ tsp basil

DIRECTIONS

1. In a bowl combine all ingredients together and mix well
2. In a skillet heat olive oil and pour the egg mixture
3. Cook for 1-2 minutes per side

4. When ready remove omelette from the skillet and
    serve

Serves: **1**

Prep Time: **5** Minutes

Cook Time: **10** Minutes

Total Time: **15** Minutes

INGREDIENTS

- **2 eggs**
- **¼ tsp salt**
- **¼ tsp black pepper**
- **1 tablespoon olive oil**
- **¼ cup cheese**
- **¼ tsp basil**
- **1 cup asparagus**

DIRECTIONS

1. **In a bowl combine all ingredients together and mix well**
2. **In a skillet heat olive oil and pour the egg mixture**
3. **Cook for 1-2 minutes per side**

4. When ready remove omelette from the skillet and
    serve

Serves: *1*

Prep Time: *5* Minutes

Cook Time: *10* Minutes

Total Time: *15* Minutes

INGREDIENTS

- 2 eggs
- ¼ tsp salt
- ¼ tsp black pepper
- 1 tablespoon olive oil
- ¼ cup cheese
- ¼ tsp basil
- 1 cup red onion
- 1 cup black beans

DIRECTIONS

1. In a bowl combine all ingredients together and mix well
2. In a skillet heat olive oil and pour the egg mixture

3. Cook for 1-2 minutes per side

4. When ready remove omelette from the skillet and
   serve

Serves: *1*

Prep Time: *5*   Minutes

Cook Time: *10*   Minutes

Total Time: *15*   Minutes

INGREDIENTS

- 2 eggs
- ¼ tsp salt
- ¼ tsp black pepper
- 1 tablespoon olive oil
- ¼ cup cheese
- ¼ tsp basil
- 1 cup lentils

DIRECTIONS

1. In a bowl combine all ingredients together and mix well
2. In a skillet heat olive oil and pour the egg mixture
3. Cook for 1-2 minutes per side

4. When ready remove omelette from the skillet and
    serve

Serves: *1*

Prep Time: *5*   Minutes

Cook Time: *10*   Minutes

Total Time: *15*   Minutes

INGREDIENTS

- **2 eggs**
- **¼ tsp salt**
- **¼ tsp black pepper**
- **1 tablespoon olive oil**
- **¼ cup cheese**
- **¼ tsp basil**
- **1 cup endive**

DIRECTIONS

1. **In a bowl combine all ingredients together and mix well**
2. **In a skillet heat olive oil and pour the egg mixture**
3. **Cook for 1-2 minutes per side**

4. When ready remove omelette from the skillet and
    serve

Serves: *1*
Prep Time: *5*   Minutes

Cook Time: *5*   Minutes

Total Time: *10*   Minutes

INGREDIENTS

- ½ cup berries
- 1 cup oats
- 1 tsp chia seeds
- 1 tablespoon flax seeds
- ¼ tsp cinnamon
- ¼ cup coconut milk

DIRECTIONS

1. In a bowl combine all ingredients together
2. Cover and refrigerate overnight
3. Serve in the morning

Serves: **6-8**

Prep Time: **5**   Minutes

Cook Time: **10**   Minutes

Total Time: **15**   Minutes

INGREDIENTS

- 1 cup pitted dates
- 1 oz. cocoa powder
- 3 oz. chia seeds
- ¼ cup coconut flakes
- 3 oz. chocolate
- 1 tsp vanilla extract
- ½ cup honey

DIRECTIONS

1. Place all the ingredients in a blender and blend until smooth
2. Remove mixture from the blender and place mixture into a baking pan
3. Press the mixture and refrigerate overnight

4. Next morning, cut into bars and serve

Serves: *1*
Prep Time: **5**   Minutes

Cook Time: **5**   Minutes

Total Time: **10**   Minutes

INGREDIENTS

- ½ banana
- ¼ cup berries
- ¼ cup watermelon
- ¼ cup almonds
- 2 tablespoons raisins
- 2 tablespoons honey

DIRECTIONS

1. In a bowl combine all ingredients together
2. Add honey and mix well
3. Serve when ready

Serves: *1*
Prep Time: *5*   Minutes

Cook Time: *10*   Minutes

Total Time: *15*   Minutes

INGREDIENTS

- 1 banana
- ¼ cup raspberries
- ¼ cup blueberries
- 1 tablespoon maple syrup

Toppings
- 1 tablespoon chia seeds
- 1 tsp hemp seeds
- 1 cup protein powder

DIRECTIONS

1. In a bowl combine all ingredients together
2. Add toppings and mix well
3. Serve when ready

Serves: **1**
Prep Time: **5** Minutes

Cook Time: **5** Minutes

Total Time: **10** Minutes

INGREDIENTS

- 1 cup water
- 2 tablespoons maple syrup
- ½ cup almond milk
- ½ cup almonds
- ¼ cup Greek yogurt

DIRECTIONS

1. Place all ingredients in a bowl and mix well
2. Refrigerate overnight
3. Serve in the morning

SIMPLE PIZZA RECIPE

Serves: **6-8**
Prep Time: **10**   Minutes

Cook Time: **15**   Minutes

Total Time: **25**   Minutes

INGREDIENTS

- 1 pizza crust
- ½ cup tomato sauce
- ¼ black pepper
- 1 cup pepperoni slices
- 1 cup mozzarella cheese
- 1 cup olives

DIRECTIONS

1. Spread tomato sauce on the pizza crust
2. Place all the toppings on the pizza crust
3. Bake the pizza at 425 F for 12-15 minutes

4. When ready remove pizza from the oven and
    serve

Serves: *6-8*
Prep Time: *10*   Minutes

Cook Time: *15*   Minutes

Total Time: *25*   Minutes

INGREDIENTS

- 1 pizza crust
- ½ cup tomato sauce
- ¼ black pepper
- 1 cup zucchini slices
- 1 cup mozzarella cheese
- 1 cup olives

DIRECTIONS

1. Spread tomato sauce on the pizza crust
2. Place all the toppings on the pizza crust
3. Bake the pizza at 425 F for 12-15 minutes
4. When ready remove pizza from the oven and serve

Serves: *2*

Prep Time: *10*   Minutes

Cook Time: *20*   Minutes

Total Time: *30*   Minutes

INGREDIENTS

- ½ lb. cabbage
- 1 tablespoon olive oil
- ½ red onion
- 2 eggs
- ¼ tsp salt
- 2 oz. cheddar cheese
- 1 garlic clove
- ¼ tsp dill

DIRECTIONS

1. In a bowl whisk eggs with salt and cheese
2. In a frying pan heat olive oil and pour egg mixture

3. Add remaining ingredients and mix well
4. Serve when ready

Serves: *2*

Prep Time: *10*   Minutes

Cook Time: *20*   Minutes

Total Time: *30*   Minutes

INGREDIENTS

- ½ lb. Brussel sprouts
- 1 tablespoon olive oil
- ½ red onion
- ¼ tsp salt
- 2 eggs
- 2 oz. cheddar cheese
- 1 garlic clove
- ¼ tsp dill

DIRECTIONS

1. In a skillet sauté Brussel sprouts until tender
2. In a bowl whisk eggs with salt and cheese

3. In a frying pan heat olive oil and pour egg
    mixture

4. Add remaining ingredients and mix well

5. Serve when ready

Serves: *2*
Prep Time: *10*   Minutes

Cook Time: *20*   Minutes

Total Time: *30*   Minutes

INGREDIENTS

- 1 cup celery
- 1 tablespoon olive oil
- ½ red onion
- ¼ tsp salt
- 2 eggs
- 2 oz. cheddar cheese
- 1 garlic clove
- ¼ tsp dill

DIRECTIONS

1. In a bowl whisk eggs with salt and cheese
2. In a frying pan heat olive oil and pour egg mixture

3. Add remaining ingredients and mix well

4. When ready serve with sautéed celery

Serves: **2**

Prep Time: **10**   Minutes

Cook Time: **20**   Minutes

Total Time: **30**   Minutes

INGREDIENTS

- **8-10 slices prosciutto**
- **1 tsp rosemary**
- **1 tablespoon olive oil**
- **½ red onion**
- **¼ tsp salt**
- **2 eggs**
- **2 oz. parmesan cheese**
- **1 garlic clove**
- **¼ tsp dill**

DIRECTIONS

1. **In a bowl whisk eggs with salt and parmesan cheese**

2. In a frying pan heat olive oil and pour egg
    mixture

3. Add remaining ingredients and mix well

4. When prosciutto and eggs are cooked remove
    from heat and serve

Serves: *2*
Prep Time: *10*   Minutes

Cook Time: *20*   Minutes

Total Time: *30*   Minutes

INGREDIENTS

- 1 tsp oregano
- 1 tablespoon olive oil
- ½ red onion
- ¼ tsp salt
- 2 eggs
- 2 oz. cheddar cheese
- 1 garlic clove
- ¼ tsp dill

DIRECTIONS

1. In a bowl whisk eggs with salt and cheese
2. In a frying pan heat olive oil and pour egg mixture

3. Add remaining ingredients and mix well
4. Serve when ready

Serves: 2
Prep Time: 5   Minutes

Cook Time: 5   Minutes

Total Time: 10   Minutes

INGREDIENTS

- 1 cup cooked brown rice
- 1 gluten-free tortilla
- 2-3 tablespoons hummus
- ¼ cup black beans
- ¼ cup tomatoes
- ¼ cup cucumber
- ¼ cup avocado
- ¼ cup romaine lettuce

DIRECTIONS

1. Microwave the tortilla for 20-30 seconds
2. Spread hummus on tortilla

3. Add beans, tomatoes, cucumber, and remaining ingredients

4. Roll like a burrito and serve

Serves: **4-6**

Prep Time: **10**   Minutes

Cook Time: **30**   Minutes

Total Time: **40**   Minutes

INGREDIENTS

- 2 white potatoes
- 1 tsp olive oil
- 1 tsp garlic powder
- 1 tsp onion powder
- salt
- 1 cup avocado dip

DIRECTIONS

1. Slice potatoes into thick slices
2. In a bowl combine garlic powder, onion powder, salt, olive oil and mix well
3. Place the potatoes into the mixture and stir to coat
4. Bake the potatoes at 425 F for 25-30 minutes

5. When ready remove from the oven and serve
    with avocado dip

Serves: *4*

Prep Time: *10*   Minutes

Cook Time: *15*   Minutes

Total Time: *25*   Minutes

INGREDIENTS

- 2 cups kale
- 1 tablespoon avocado oil
- 1 tsp salt
- 1 tsp turmeric
- 1 tsp chili powder
- 1 tsp curry powder

DIRECTIONS

1. In a bowl combine all ingredients except kale
2. Mix well and add kale to the seasoning mixture
3. Toss to coat and then place the kale in a baking dish
4. Bake at 250 F for 12-15 minutes

5. **When ready remove from the oven and serve**

60

Serves: **2**
Prep Time: **10**   Minutes

Cook Time: **20**   Minutes

Total Time: **30**   Minutes

INGREDIENTS

- 1 tablespoon olive oil
- 1 clove garlic
- 1 lb. pork
- ½ red onion
- 1 cup carrot
- 1 cabbage
- ½ cup soy sauce
- ¼ tsp black pepper

DIRECTIONS

1. In a skillet sauté garlic and onion until soft
2. Add pork, cabbage and cook for another 6-7 minutes

3. Add soy sauce, carrot and cook until vegetables
    are tender

4. When ready transfer mixture to a bowl, add
    pepper and serve

Serves: *1*

Prep Time: *10* Minutes

Cook Time: *20* Minutes

Total Time: *30* Minutes

INGREDIENTS

- 1 tablespoon olive oil
- 1 chicken breast
- 1 tsp oregano
- 1 tsp black pepper
- 1 cup tomatoes
- ¼ cucumber
- ¼ cup red onion
- ¼ cup black olives
- 1/4 cup feta cheese
- 1 cup dressing

DIRECTIONS

1. In a skillet add chicken and cook until golden

2. Add seasoning and onion

3. When ready place all ingredients in a bowl

4. Drizzle dressing on top, mix well and serve

Serves: **2**

Prep Time: **5** Minutes

Cook Time: **5** Minutes

Total Time: **10** Minutes

INGREDIENTS

- **1 can unsweetened pineapple**
- **1 package cherry gelatin**
- **1 tablespoon lemon juice**
- **½ cup artificial sweetener**
- **1 cup cranberries**
- **1 orange**
- **1 cup celery**
- **½ cup pecans**

DIRECTIONS

1. **In a bowl mix all ingredients and mix well**
2. **Serve with dressing**

Serves: **2**
Prep Time: **5**   Minutes

Cook Time: **5**   Minutes

Total Time: **10**   Minutes

INGREDIENTS

- 1 cup broccoli
- 1 cup quinoa
- 2 radishes
- 2 tablespoons pumpkin seeds
- 1 cup salad dressing

DIRECTIONS

1. In a bowl mix all ingredients and mix well
2. Serve with dressing

Serves: **2**

Prep Time: **5**   Minutes

Cook Time: **5**   Minutes

Total Time: ***10***   Minutes

INGREDIENTS

- 2 carrots
- 2 purple carrots
- 1 cabbage
- ¼ red onion
- 1 bunch leaves
- 2 kale leaves
- 1 cup salad dressing

DIRECTIONS

1. In a bowl mix all ingredients and mix well
2. Serve with dressing

Serves: **2**

Prep Time: **5**   Minutes

Cook Time: **5**   Minutes

Total Time: **10**   Minutes

INGREDIENTS

- **1 lb. broad beans**
- **½ lb. peas**
- **2 chives**
- **Mint leaves**
- **2 spring onions**
- **2 tablespoons olive oil**
- **2 tablespoons lemon juice**

DIRECTIONS

1. **In a bowl mix all ingredients and mix well**
2. **Serve with dressing**

Serves: **2**

Prep Time: **5**   Minutes

Cook Time: **5**   Minutes

Total Time: **10**   Minutes

INGREDIENTS

- 1 bunch coriander leaves
- 1 bunch mint leaves
- ¼ red onion
- 1 bunch parsley
- 1 cup lentils
- 1 tablespoon pumpkin seeds
- 1 tablespoon pine nuts

DIRECTIONS

1. In a bowl mix all ingredients and mix well
2. Serve with dressing

Serves: **2**
Prep Time: **5**   Minutes

Cook Time: **5**   Minutes

Total Time: **10**   Minutes

INGREDIENTS

- 1 cauliflower
- 4 slices bacon
- ¼ cup sour cream
- ¼ cup mayonnaise
- 1 tablespoon lemon juice
- ¼ tsp garlic powder
- 1 cup cheddar cheese
- ¼ cup chives

DIRECTIONS

1. In a bowl mix all ingredients and mix well
2. Serve with dressing

Serves: 2
Prep Time: 5   Minutes

Cook Time: 5   Minutes

Total Time: *10*   Minutes

INGREDIENTS

- 1 cup buffalo sauce
- 1 tablespoon lime juice
- 1 tsp garlic powder
- ¼ tsp onion powder
- 1 lb. cooked chicken breast
- 1 tablespoon olive oil

DIRECTIONS

1. In a bowl mix all ingredients and mix well
2. Serve with dressing

Serves: **2**

Prep Time: **5**   Minutes

Cook Time: **5**   Minutes

Total Time: **10**   Minutes

INGREDIENTS

- **1 lb. carrots**
- **¼ cup raisins**
- **¼ cup peanuts**
- **¼ cup cilantro**
- **2 green onions**
- **¼ cup olive oil**
- **1 tablespoon honey**
- **1 tablespoon lime juice**
- **1 tsp cumin**

DIRECTIONS

1. **In a bowl mix all ingredients and mix well**
2. **Serve with dressing**

Serves: *2*

Prep Time: *5*   Minutes

Cook Time: *5*   Minutes

Total Time: *10*   Minutes

INGREDIENTS

- 1 cup cooked FARRO
- 1 bay leaf
- 1 shallot
- ¼ cup olive oil
- 1 tablespoon apple cider vinegar
- 2 cups arugula
- ¼ cup parmesan cheese
- ¼ cup basil
- ¼ cup parsley
- ¼ cup pecans

DIRECTIONS

1. In a bowl mix all ingredients and mix well

2. Serve with dressing

Serves: **2**

Prep Time: **5**   Minutes

Cook Time: **5**   Minutes

Total Time: **10**   Minutes

INGREDIENTS

- **2 cups corn**
- **2 cups tomatoes**
- **¼ cup feta**
- **¼ red onion**
- **¼ cup basil**
- **2 tablespoons olive oil**
- **Juice of ½ lime**

DIRECTIONS

1. **In a bowl mix all ingredients and mix well**
2. **Serve with dressing**

CAULIFLOWER RECIPE

Serves: **6-8**
Prep Time: **10**   Minutes

Cook Time: **15**   Minutes

Total Time: **25**   Minutes

INGREDIENTS

- 1 pizza crust
- ½ cup tomato sauce
- ¼ black pepper
- 1 cup cauliflower
- 1 cup mozzarella cheese
- 1 cup olives

DIRECTIONS

1. Spread tomato sauce on the pizza crust
2. Place all the toppings on the pizza crust
3. Bake the pizza at 425 F for 12-15 minutes

4. When ready remove pizza from the oven and
    serve

Serves: *6-8*
Prep Time: *10*   Minutes

Cook Time: *15*   Minutes

Total Time: *25*   Minutes

INGREDIENTS

- 1 pizza crust
- ½ cup tomato sauce
- ¼ black pepper
- 1 cup broccoli
- 1 cup mozzarella cheese
- 1 cup olives

DIRECTIONS

1. Spread tomato sauce on the pizza crust
2. Place all the toppings on the pizza crust
3. Bake the pizza at 425 F for 12-15 minutes
4. When ready remove pizza from the oven and serve

Serves: **6-8**

Prep Time: **10** Minutes

Cook Time: **15** Minutes

Total Time: **25** Minutes

INGREDIENTS

- 1 pizza crust
- ½ cup tomato sauce
- ¼ black pepper
- 1 cup pepperoni slices
- 1 cup tomatoes
- 6-8 ham slices
- 1 cup mozzarella cheese
- 1 cup olives

DIRECTIONS

1. Spread tomato sauce on the pizza crust
2. Place all the toppings on the pizza crust
3. Bake the pizza at 425 F for 12-15 minutes

4. When ready remove pizza from the oven and
    serve

Serves: **4**

Prep Time: **10**   Minutes

Cook Time: **20**   Minutes

Total Time: **30**   Minutes

INGREDIENTS

- 1 tablespoon olive oil
- 1 lb. mushrooms
- ¼ red onion
- ½ cup all-purpose flour
- ¼ tsp salt
- ¼ tsp pepper
- 1 can vegetable broth
- 1 cup heavy cream

DIRECTIONS

1. In a saucepan heat olive oil and sauté mushrooms until tender
2. Add remaining ingredients to the saucepan and bring to a boil

3. When all the vegetables are tender transfer to a blender and blend until smooth

4. Pour soup into bowls, garnish with parsley and serve

Serves: **4**

Prep Time: **10**   Minutes

Cook Time: **20**   Minutes

Total Time: **30**   Minutes

INGREDIENTS

- 1 tablespoon olive oil
- 1 lb. zucchini
- ¼ red onion
- ½ cup all-purpose flour
- ¼ tsp salt
- ¼ tsp pepper
- 1 can vegetable broth
- 1 cup heavy cream

DIRECTIONS

1. In a saucepan heat olive oil and sauté zucchini until tender

5. Add remaining ingredients to the saucepan and bring to a boil

6. When all the vegetables are tender transfer to a
    blender and blend until smooth

7. Pour soup into bowls, garnish with parsley and
    serve

Serves: *4*

Prep Time: *10*   Minutes

Cook Time: *20*   Minutes

Total Time: *30*   Minutes

INGREDIENTS

- **1 tablespoon olive oil**
- **1 lb. spinach**
- **¼ red onion**
- **½ cup all-purpose flour**
- **¼ tsp salt**
- **¼ tsp pepper**
- **1 can vegetable broth**
- **1 cup heavy cream**

DIRECTIONS

1. **In a saucepan heat olive oil and sauté spinach until tender**
2. **Add remaining ingredients to the saucepan and bring to a boil**

3. When all the vegetables are tender transfer to a blender and blend until smooth

4. Pour soup into bowls, garnish with parsley and serve

Serves: **4**

Prep Time: **10**   Minutes

Cook Time: **20**   Minutes

Total Time: **30**   Minutes

INGREDIENTS

- 1 tablespoon olive oil
- 1 lb. carrots
- ¼ red onion
- ½ cup all-purpose flour
- ¼ tsp salt
- ¼ tsp pepper
- 1 can vegetable broth
- 1 cup heavy cream

DIRECTIONS

1. In a saucepan heat olive oil and sauté carrots until tender
2. Add remaining ingredients to the saucepan and bring to a boil

3. When all the vegetables are tender transfer to a blender and blend until smooth

4. Pour soup into bowls, garnish with parsley and serve

Serves: **4**

Prep Time: **10**   Minutes

Cook Time: **20**   Minutes

Total Time: **30**   Minutes

INGREDIENTS

- 1 tablespoon olive oil
- 1 lb. mushrooms
- ¼ red onion
- ½ cup all-purpose flour
- ¼ tsp salt
- ¼ tsp pepper
- 1 can vegetable broth
- 1 cup heavy cream

DIRECTIONS

1. In a saucepan heat olive oil and sauté potatoes until tender
2. Add remaining ingredients to the saucepan and bring to a boil

3. When all the vegetables are tender transfer to a blender and blend until smooth

4. Pour soup into bowls, garnish with parsley and serve

OMBRE SMOOTHIE

Serves: *1*
Prep Time: *5*   Minutes

Cook Time: *5*   Minutes

Total Time: *10*   Minutes

INGREDIENTS

- 1 pineapple
- 1 mango
- 1 cup water
- 1 cup raspberries

DIRECTIONS

1. In a blender place all ingredients and blend until smooth
2. Pour smoothie in a glass and serve

Serves: *1*
Prep Time: *5*   Minutes

Cook Time: *5*   Minutes

Total Time: *10*   Minutes

INGREDIENTS

- 1 cup milk
- 3 oz. Greek Yogurt
- 1 tsp vanilla essence
- 1 banana
- ½ papaya
- 1 cup ice

DIRECTIONS

1. In a blender place all ingredients and blend until smooth
2. Pour smoothie in a glass and serve

Serves: *1*
Prep Time: **5**   Minutes

Cook Time: **5**   Minutes

Total Time: ***10***   Minutes

INGREDIENTS

- 2 pears
- 1 tsp chia seeds
- 1 pear
- 1 pinch cinnamon

DIRECTIONS

1. **In a blender place all ingredients and blend until smooth**
2. **Pour smoothie in a glass and serve**

Serves: *1*
Prep Time: **5**   Minutes

Cook Time: **5**   Minutes

Total Time: *10*   Minutes

INGREDIENTS

- 1 cup berries
- 1 banana
- ½ cup orange juice
- 1 cup ice

DIRECTIONS

1. In a blender place all ingredients and blend until smooth
2. Pour smoothie in a glass and serve

Serves: *1*
Prep Time: *5*   Minutes

Cook Time: *5*   Minutes

Total Time: *10*   Minutes

INGREDIENTS

- 2 avocados
- ¼ cup spinach
- 1 apple
- 1 kiwi
- 1 cup ice
- ½ cup water

DIRECTIONS

1. In a blender place all ingredients and blend until smooth
2. Pour smoothie in a glass and serve

Serves: *1*
Prep Time: **5**   Minutes

Cook Time: **5**   Minutes

Total Time: **10**   Minutes

INGREDIENTS

- 1 cup oats
- ¼ cup raisins
- ¼ tsp pumpkin pie
- 1 cup milk
- ¼ cup vanilla yoghurt

DIRECTIONS

1. In a blender place all ingredients and blend until smooth
2. Pour smoothie in a glass and serve

Serves: *1*
Prep Time: *5*   Minutes

Cook Time: *5*   Minutes

Total Time: *10*   Minutes

INGREDIENTS

- 2 cups peaches
- 1 cup apricots
- 1 banana
- 1 cup milk
- 1 tsp vanilla extract
- 1 tablespoon mint
- 1 cup ice
- Mint leaves

DIRECTIONS

1. In a blender place all ingredients and blend until smooth
2. Pour smoothie in a glass and serve

Serves: *1*
Prep Time: *5*   Minutes

Cook Time: *5*   Minutes

Total Time: *10*   Minutes

INGREDIENTS

- **2 oz. soy milk**
- **2 oz. acai**
- **1 banana**
- **5 oz. strawberries**
- **5 oz. blueberries**

DIRECTIONS

1. **In a blender place all ingredients and blend until smooth**
2. **Pour smoothie in a glass and serve**

Serves: *1*
Prep Time: *5*   Minutes

Cook Time: *5*   Minutes

Total Time: *10*   Minutes

INGREDIENTS

- 4 strawberries
- ½ cup watermelon
- ½ cup peaches
- 2 scoops raspberries
- 2 oz. orange juice

DIRECTIONS

1. In a blender place all ingredients and blend until smooth
2. Pour smoothie in a glass and serve

Serves: *1*
Prep Time: *5*   Minutes

Cook Time: *5*   Minutes

Total Time: *10*   Minutes

INGREDIENTS

- 1 cup orange juice
- 2 oz. lime juice
- ½ cup strawberries
- 1 banana

DIRECTIONS

1. In a blender place all ingredients and blend until smooth
2. Pour smoothie in a glass and serve

THANK YOU FOR READING THIS BOOK!